# DEMENTIA REFLECTIONS

*Showing Love and Care to People Living with Dementia*

**NANCY JUDY**

# COPYRIGHT

Copyright © 2024 by Nancy Judy: All rights reserved. This book or any portion thereof may not be reproduced or used in any manner whatsoever without the express written permission of the author except for the use of brief quotations in a book review.

# TABLE OF CONTENTS

ABOUT THE BOOK .................................................................................................... 5

INTRODUCTION ....................................................................................................... 7
    NAVIGATING THE HEART AND SOUL OF DEMENTIA CARE ........................... 7

CHAPTER 1 .................................................................................................................. 9
    UNDERSTANDING DEMENTIA ........................................................................... 9

CHAPTER 2 ................................................................................................................ 16
    DIFFERENTIATING HALLUCINATIONS AND DELUSIONS IN DEMENTIA .... 16

CHAPTER 3 ................................................................................................................ 22
    TOOLS AND TECHNIQUES FOR MEMORY SUPPORT .................................... 22

CHAPTER 4 ................................................................................................................ 27
    EMERGENCY PREPAREDNESS: A COMPREHENSIVE GUIDE ........................ 27

CHAPTER 5 ................................................................................................................ 33
    DISTRACTION TECHNIQUES FOR CAREGIVERS ............................................ 33

CHAPTER 6 ................................................................................................................ 39
    FOSTERING STRONG CONNECTIONS WITH DEMENTIA PATIENTS ........... 39

CHAPTER 7 ................................................................................................................ 46
    CAREGIVER WELLNESS ..................................................................................... 46

CHAPTER 8 ................................................................................................................ 53
    AVOIDING CAREGIVER BURNOUT .................................................................. 53

CHAPTER 9 ................................................................................................................ 59
    FINANCIAL SAFEGUARDING ............................................................................ 59

CHAPTER 10 .............................................................................................................. 65
    ENGAGING ACTIVITIES FOR DEMENTIA PATIENTS ..................................... 65

**CONCLUSION** ........................................................................................................................... **68**
    **EMBRACING WISDOM AND HOPE** ........................................................................... **68**

# ABOUT THE BOOK

In the pages of "Dementia Reflections," readers embark on a poignant exploration of the complexities, challenges, and profound moments of grace encountered in the realm of dementia care. Written with a blend of storytelling finesse, modern language, and practical wisdom, this book serves as a compassionate guide through the labyrinthine landscape of caregiving.

**1. The Heart of Dementia Care**

Embracing Compassion: Stories illustrating the transformative power of empathy and understanding in caregiving.

Journeying Together: Insights into familial dynamics, resilience, and the bonds forged amidst adversity.

**2. Understanding Dementia**

Defining Dementia: A comprehensive overview of dementia types, symptoms, and the scientific underpinnings of the condition.

Recognizing Early Signs: Practical advice on identifying cognitive decline and proactive steps to support loved ones.

**3. Tools for Care and Connection**

Memory Support Techniques: From memory aids to technology, strategies to enhance daily life and foster meaningful interactions.

Distraction Techniques: Engaging activities and sensory approaches to alleviate stress and promote engagement.

## 4. Caregiver Wellness

Nurturing the Caregiver: Techniques for maintaining physical health, managing stress, and cultivating resilience.

Avoiding Burnout: Strategies to recognize burnout, prioritize self-care, and build a supportive network.

## 5. Financial Safeguarding

Protecting Assets: Practical tips on safeguarding finances, recognizing financial abuse, and long-term planning for dementia care.

Navigating Benefits: Insights into insurance options, government programs, and resources for financial support.

## 6. Engaging Activities for Joy and Connection

Creative Pursuits: Ideas for simple, enjoyable activities tailored to different stages of dementia.

Physical Well-being: Safe exercises and movement therapies to enhance quality of life and promote holistic wellness.

"Dementia Reflections" is not merely a guidebook but a companion—a testament to the human spirit's capacity for compassion, resilience, and growth amidst adversity. Through its pages, readers discover practical strategies, heartfelt stories, and invaluable insights that illuminate the path forward with grace and understanding in the journey with dementia.

# INTRODUCTION

In the quiet moments of caregiving, amidst the ebb and flow of memories and emotions, lies a profound journey illuminated by courage, compassion, and resilience.

Each page of this book is a reflection—a mirror that captures the complexities and realities faced by caregivers, families, and individuals navigating the terrain of dementia. It is a testament to the profound impact of empathy and understanding in the lives of those affected by this condition—where every gesture of kindness, every shared moment, becomes a thread binding hearts in a journey of care and connection.

Through storytelling that resonates with modern language and practical wisdom, "Dementia Reflections" illuminates the multifaceted dimensions of dementia care. From understanding the scientific foundations of the condition to exploring innovative tools and techniques for support, this book serves as a compassionate guide. It empowers caregivers with insights on nurturing their own well-being, navigating financial considerations, and engaging in activities that promote joy and connection.

Drawing from personal experiences and professional insights, "Dementia Reflections" seeks to uplift and inspire. It honors the resilience of caregivers and celebrates the enduring spirit of those living with dementia. More than a guidebook, it is a companion—a source of solace, guidance, and hope for anyone touched by the journey of dementia.

As you embark on this exploration of heart and soul, may "Dementia Reflections" serve as a beacon of light—a reminder that amidst the challenges, there are moments of profound beauty and connection waiting to be discovered. Together, let us navigate this journey with compassion, understanding, and unwavering dedication to enriching lives affected by dementia.

# CHAPTER 1

## UNDERSTANDING DEMENTIA

Dementia is a broad term that encompasses a range of progressive neurological disorders characterized by the decline in cognitive function severe enough to interfere with daily life and independence. This deterioration impacts memory, thinking, orientation, comprehension, calculation, learning capacity, language, and judgment. Dementia is not a single disease but a syndrome with various causes, often associated with aging, but it is not a normal part of the aging process.

Dementia is not just forgetfulness; it's a labyrinthine disorder that alters the very essence of memory and cognition. Imagine a house where the rooms, once familiar and comforting, start losing their walls, their furniture fading into obscurity. This is dementia—an umbrella term for a group of symptoms affecting memory, thinking, and social abilities severely enough to interfere with daily functioning.

**Types and Variations of Dementia**

Within this maze, there are different paths. Alzheimer's disease, the most common form of dementia, slowly erases memories like a fading photograph. Vascular dementia, often a result of strokes or other conditions affecting blood flow to the brain, disrupts cognitive function in sudden bursts. Other types, like Lewy body dementia and frontotemporal dementia, each have their unique way of distorting perception and understanding.

There are several types and variations of dementia, each with unique characteristics:

**1. Alzheimer's Disease:** The most common form, accounting for 60-80% of cases. It involves the accumulation of amyloid plaques and tau tangles in the brain, leading to neuronal damage and brain atrophy.

**2. Vascular Dementia**: Caused by conditions that block or reduce blood flow to the brain, leading to brain damage. It often results from strokes or a series of small, unnoticeable strokes.

**3. Lewy Body Dementia:** Characterized by the presence of Lewy bodies (abnormal clumps of protein) in the brain. It shares symptoms with both Alzheimer's and Parkinson's diseases, including hallucinations and movement disorders.

**4. Frontotemporal Dementia:** Involves the progressive degeneration of the frontal and temporal lobes of the brain. It affects personality, behavior, and language more than memory.

**5. Mixed Dementia:** A combination of two or more types of dementia, typically Alzheimer's disease and vascular dementia.

**6. Other Types:** Less common forms include Huntington's disease, Creutzfeldt-Jakob disease, and Wernicke-Korsakoff syndrome.

**Recognizing Dementia**

**Early Warning Signs of Cognitive Decline**

Identifying dementia early can be challenging, as the symptoms may be subtle initially and resemble normal aging. However, some early warning signs include:

**1. Memory Loss:** Particularly short-term memory loss, where recent events, names, and places are forgotten.

**2. Difficulty in Planning or Solving Problems:** Struggling to follow plans or work with numbers, such as keeping track of monthly bills.

**3. Confusion with Time or Place**: Losing track of dates, seasons, and the passage of time.

**4. Problems with Speaking or Writing:** Difficulty in following or joining conversations, or struggling to find the right words.

**5. Misplacing Things:** Putting items in unusual places and being unable to retrace steps to find them.

**6. Poor Judgment:** Experiencing changes in decision-making and judgment, such as poor financial decisions.

7. Withdrawal from Social Activities: Avoiding social interactions, work projects, or hobbies once enjoyed.

**8. Changes in Mood and Personality:** Becoming confused, suspicious, depressed, fearful, or anxious.

**Actions to Prevent the Condition from Worsening**

While there is no cure for dementia, certain actions may help slow its progression and improve quality of life:

**1. Mental Stimulation:** Engage in activities that challenge the brain, such as puzzles, reading, or learning new skills.

**2. Physical Activity:** Regular exercise can improve cardiovascular health, which in turn benefits brain health.

**3. Healthy Diet:** Consuming a balanced diet rich in fruits, vegetables, whole grains, and lean proteins can support brain function.

**4. Social Engagement:** Staying socially active helps maintain cognitive function and emotional well-being.

**5. Quality Sleep:** Ensure adequate sleep to support overall brain health.

**6. Manage Chronic Conditions:** Properly manage conditions like diabetes, hypertension, and high cholesterol.

**7. Avoid Harmful Habits:** Reduce or eliminate smoking and excessive alcohol consumption.


**The Science Behind Dementia**

**How Dementia Affects the Brain**

Inside the brain, dementia unleashes chaos. Beta-amyloid plaques accumulate, disrupting communication between neurons in Alzheimer's. In vascular dementia, clots block vital pathways, starving brain cells of oxygen. Each variant leaves its mark on the brain's intricate network, fraying the threads of memory and reason.

Dementia affects the brain in several ways, depending on the type. Common mechanisms include:

**1. Neuronal Damage and Death:** Accumulation of abnormal proteins like amyloid-beta and tau in Alzheimer's disease leads to the death of neurons.

**2. Reduced Blood Flow:** In vascular dementia, blocked or damaged blood vessels reduce blood flow, depriving brain cells of oxygen and nutrients.

**3. Protein Aggregates:** In Lewy body dementia, abnormal protein aggregates interfere with brain cell function.

**4. Lobe Degeneration:** In frontotemporal dementia, specific brain regions shrink, affecting related functions such as behavior and language.

**Current Research and Future Directions**

The scientific community is actively researching to better understand and combat dementia. Some promising directions include:

**1. Biomarker Identification:** Finding biomarkers for early detection, allowing for earlier intervention and monitoring.

**2. Genetic Research:** Investigating genetic factors that contribute to dementia to develop targeted therapies.

**3. Neuroimaging:** Advanced imaging techniques to visualize brain changes and track disease progression.

**4. Drug Development:** Exploring new medications to slow or halt the progression of dementia. Recent advancements include drugs targeting amyloid plaques and tau tangles.

**5. Lifestyle Interventions:** Research into how diet, exercise, and cognitive training can mitigate dementia risk and progression.

Imagine a bustling city as a metaphor for the brain. In a healthy brain, like a well-functioning city, there are seamless connections, smooth communication, and efficient operation of all its parts. Now, picture this city facing a series of disruptive events – roads blocked by fallen trees (representing amyloid plaques), traffic lights malfunctioning (tau tangles), and reduced fuel supply to power its activities (vascular issues). Over time, these disruptions cause chaos, confusion, and gradual deterioration of the city's functionality.

John, a retired schoolteacher, once prided himself on his sharp memory and vibrant social life. He loved recounting tales of his travels and engaging in lively debates. But gradually, John noticed small lapses – forgetting a friend's name or losing track of his favorite book. His family observed his growing frustration and decided to seek medical advice. Early intervention helped John manage his condition better, and with a combination of medication, cognitive exercises, and a supportive environment, he continued to share his stories, albeit with a few gaps.

Dementia is a journey into the unknown—a journey that millions embark on each year, their paths intertwining with those who care for them. Understanding dementia means embracing its complexities with empathy and knowledge, seeking not just to navigate its challenges but to illuminate the way forward. In this quest, science and humanity converge, offering hope and determination in equal measure.

In laboratories around the world, scientists are racing against time, probing the mysteries of dementia. From genetic predispositions to environmental triggers, every clue holds promise. Advances in imaging technology allow glimpses into the brain's inner workings, while clinical trials explore new treatments and therapies. The hope is not just to slow dementia's advance but to one day prevent it altogether.

If you or a loved one is experiencing signs of dementia, it's crucial to seek medical advice promptly. Early diagnosis can lead to better management and improved quality of life. Maintain a healthy lifestyle, stay mentally and socially active, and never hesitate to reach out for support. Remember, while dementia poses significant challenges, understanding and proactive care can make a meaningful difference.

# CHAPTER 2

## DIFFERENTIATING HALLUCINATIONS AND DELUSIONS IN DEMENTIA

Understanding the distinctions between hallucinations and delusions is crucial for effectively managing dementia patients, as these symptoms significantly impact their well-being and care.

**Hallucinations in Dementia**

Hallucinations are false sensory perceptions that occur without an external stimulus. In other words, the person experiences something that isn't actually there. These can involve any of the senses, but visual and auditory hallucinations are the most common. For instance, a person might see things that others cannot see or hear voices that others cannot hear.

Hallucinations are like unexpected guests in the mind's theater—perceptions that seem real but are not grounded in external reality. For those with dementia, these sensory intrusions can take many forms: seeing people who aren't there, hearing voices, or even feeling sensations that have no physical basis. It's as if the boundaries between imagination and reality blur, casting shadows where there should be light.

**Common Causes of Hallucinations in Dementia Patients**

In the labyrinth of dementia, hallucinations often arise from the brain's struggle to process sensory information. Neurological changes, medication side effects, and sensory deprivation—all can contribute to these vivid experiences. For instance, a person with Alzheimer's might see a long-deceased loved one, their brain conjuring memories like ghosts in the fog of forgetting.

**1. Lewy Body Dementia (LBD):** Hallucinations are particularly prevalent in LBD. Patients may see vivid images of people or animals.

**2. Alzheimer's Disease:** In later stages, Alzheimer's can cause hallucinations due to severe brain changes.

**3. Parkinson's Disease Dementia:** Similar to LBD, Parkinson's can lead to visual hallucinations.

**4. Medications:** Some medications, particularly those used to treat Parkinson's, can induce hallucinations as a side effect.

**5. Sensory Deprivation:** Hearing or vision loss can contribute to hallucinations because the brain may misinterpret signals.

**Case Studies and Real-Life Examples**

**Case Study 1: Mrs. Thompson's Imaginary Children**

**Mrs. Thompson, an 82-year-old woman with advanced** Alzheimer's, often sees children playing in her living room. She sometimes offers them snacks and scolds them for being noisy. Her family learned to gently acknowledge her experiences without affirming the hallucinations, helping her feel safe without reinforcing the false perceptions.

**Case Study 2: Mr. Harris and the Phantom Cat**

Mr. Harris, a 75-year-old man with Lewy Body Dementia, frequently sees a cat sitting on his bed. Initially, his caregivers tried to convince him that the cat wasn't real, which agitated him. They later adopted a more supportive approach by calmly talking to him about the cat, which reduced his distress.

**Delusions in Dementia**

Delusions, unlike hallucinations, are fixed beliefs that defy reason and evidence. In dementia, these beliefs can be elaborate and persistent: accusing loved ones of theft, believing oneself to be in imminent danger, or even asserting a new identity altogether. Delusions weave intricate narratives, anchoring the person in a distorted reality that feels unquestionably true to them.

Delusions are strongly held false beliefs that are resistant to reason or contrary evidence. Unlike hallucinations, delusions are cognitive and not sensory. For example, a person might believe that their spouse is an impostor or that someone is stealing from them.

**Differences Between Delusions and Hallucinations**

- Nature of Experience: Hallucinations involve the senses and the perception of things that are not present, whereas delusions involve false beliefs and ideas.
- Response to Reality: Delusions are beliefs and can be complex, often involving elaborate narratives. Hallucinations are sensory experiences and may not have a narrative structure.

- Management Approach: Hallucinations might be managed by adjusting sensory input or environment, while delusions often require reassurance and cognitive interventions.

**Strategies to Manage Delusions**

**1. Validation Therapy:** Acknowledge the person's feelings without confirming the delusion. For instance, if someone believes their wallet was stolen, say, "I can see you're worried about your wallet. Let's look for it together."

**2. Redirect Attention:** Shift the person's focus to a different activity to divert their mind from the delusion.

**3. Maintain Calm Environment:** Reducing stressors in the environment can help decrease the frequency of delusions.

**4. Medication:** In some cases, antipsychotic medications may be necessary, but these should be used cautiously due to potential side effects.

**Communication Techniques**

**How to Talk to Someone Experiencing Hallucinations or Delusions**

Effective communication is vital when interacting with someone experiencing hallucinations or delusions. Communication becomes a lifeline in the fog of dementia, where words carry weight beyond their literal meaning. When faced with hallucinations or delusions, validating emotions while gently redirecting the conversation can anchor reality without denying the person's experience. For instance, if someone insists on seeing a visitor who isn't there, acknowledging their perception ("It sounds like you're seeing someone") before gently changing the subject ("Let's talk about something else you enjoy"). Here are some techniques:

- Stay Calm and Supportive: Maintain a calm demeanor. Your calmness can help reduce the person's anxiety and agitation.

- Do Not Argue: Avoid trying to convince the person that their hallucination or delusion is not real. This can increase their distress.

- Use Simple Language: Clear, simple, and direct language is easier for dementia patients to understand.

- Provide Reassurance: Offer comfort and reassurance. For instance, "I am here with you, and you are safe."

**Language and Tone Tips for Caregivers**

The language we use shapes the reality we inhabit together. Choosing calm, reassuring tones and avoiding confrontation or contradicting the person's reality can reduce distress. Simple, concrete language helps maintain clarity, while non-verbal cues—like a comforting touch or a smile—convey understanding beyond words.

- Empathy and Understanding: Use empathetic language to show you understand their feelings. "It must be scary to see those things. I'm here with you."
- Non-Threatening Tone: Keep your tone neutral and non-threatening. Avoid raising your voice or showing frustration.

- Body Language: Use positive body language, like maintaining eye contact and gentle touches, to convey reassurance.
- Storytelling Elements: Sometimes, incorporating storytelling can help. For instance, if the person is seeing a nonexistent cat, you might say, "That reminds me of a cat I once had. Let's talk about it."

**Practical Advice**

**1. Prepare the Environment:** Ensure the living space is safe and comfortable, with adequate lighting and minimal clutter.

**2. Routine and Consistency:** Maintain a consistent daily routine to provide structure and reduce confusion.

**3. Engage in Activities:** Encourage participation in simple activities that the person enjoys, which can divert their attention from hallucinations or delusions.

**4. Seek Professional Help:** Regularly consult healthcare professionals for advice and medication management.

Understanding and effectively responding to hallucinations and delusions in dementia patients require a blend of empathy, practical strategies, and consistent communication techniques. By employing these approaches, caregivers can create a supportive environment that enhances the quality of life for those affected by dementia.

# CHAPTER 3

## TOOLS AND TECHNIQUES FOR MEMORY SUPPORT

In the heart of a bustling city, there lived a woman named Margaret who was determined to keep her mind as sharp as ever. Having watched her mother struggle with dementia, Margaret sought to understand how she could protect her own cognitive health. This journey led her to discover the invaluable Dementia Risk Checklist.

**Identifying Risk Factors**

The checklist began with identifying risk factors that could increase the likelihood of developing dementia. Margaret learned that age was a significant factor—most individuals diagnosed with dementia were over 65. However, she also discovered that genetics played a role; a family history of dementia could elevate her risk.

Other risk factors included lifestyle choices and health conditions. Margaret noted that smoking, excessive alcohol consumption, and a sedentary lifestyle could all contribute to cognitive decline. Additionally, health issues like hypertension, diabetes, and high cholesterol were flagged as important concerns.

Imagine a compass guiding you through the currents of memory—a dementia risk checklist that helps chart potential dangers ahead. Age, family history, cardiovascular health—each factor casts its shadow on the path, warning of possible bends in the road. Identifying these risks early empowers individuals and caregivers to navigate with foresight.

**How to Use the Checklist Effectively**

Margaret realized that simply knowing these risk factors wasn't enough; she needed to take proactive steps. The checklist provided practical advice on how to mitigate these risks. For instance, it recommended regular physical activity, a balanced diet rich in fruits and vegetables, and maintaining a healthy weight.

Margaret also found sections on mental stimulation and social engagement. The checklist suggested activities like reading, solving puzzles, and staying socially active to keep her brain engaged. By systematically going through the checklist and making necessary lifestyle adjustments, Margaret felt more empowered to take control of her cognitive health.

**Memory Aids**

Margaret's friend, George, was a retired school teacher who had begun to notice his memory slipping. Determined to stay independent, George explored various **memory aids** that could support his daily life.

**Using Memory Boards, Memory Books, and Flashcards**

- Memory aids are like signposts in the fog, guiding thoughts back to familiar shores. For James, who battled Alzheimer's, a memory board adorned with photos and reminders became a lifeline. Each picture, each note—a thread weaving through the labyrinth of forgetting, anchoring him to cherished memories.

- George discovered that "memory boards"—large, visible boards where he could write reminders, daily schedules, and important tasks—helped him stay organized. Each morning, he would update his memory board, ensuring he wouldn't forget essential appointments or errands.

- He also started using "memory books". These were personalized photo albums filled with pictures of family members, friends, and significant events from his past. Beside each photo, George wrote brief notes to remind him of names, places, and memories associated with them. Flipping through his memory book brought back warm memories and helped him stay connected with his personal history.
- "Flashcards" became another valuable tool. George used them to reinforce the names of new acquaintances, vocabulary from the books he read, and even for practicing new skills he wanted to learn. The repetitive nature of flashcards helped solidify information in his mind.

**How to Create Personalized Memory Aids**

Creating these aids is an art of empathy and creativity. Personalized memory books with anecdotes and photographs that tell a story—a life encapsulated in pages. Flashcards, too, can be tailored to individual interests and routines, each card a beacon of familiarity in the sea of uncertainty.

Creating these aids required some creativity and personalization. George's daughter helped him by gathering family photos and writing detailed captions for the memory book. For the memory board, they bought colorful markers and sticky notes to make it more engaging. When creating flashcards, George focused on areas where he felt his memory was weakest, ensuring the aids were tailored to his specific needs.

**Technology and Dementia**

As Margaret and George continued to explore ways to support their memory, they discovered the potential of modern technology. Their neighbor, Lisa, introduced them to various "apps and devices" designed to assist with memory.

**Apps and Devices that Can Assist with Memory**

Lisa recommended a few standout apps, such as "Lumosity" and "CogniFit", which offered brain training exercises tailored to improve cognitive function. These apps provided fun and engaging activities that challenged their minds daily.

For practical day-to-day support, Lisa suggested "Reminders" and "Google Calendar" apps. These tools allowed them to set up reminders for medication, appointments, and important tasks, ensuring they never missed a beat.

Devices like "Amazon Echo" and "Google Home" became their new companions. These voice-activated assistants could set reminders, answer questions, and even provide entertainment, making their lives more manageable and enjoyable.

**Pros and Cons of Technological Aids**

However, technology came with its own set of challenges. Margaret appreciated the convenience but sometimes felt overwhelmed by the complexity of new devices. George, who wasn't as tech-savvy, struggled initially to navigate the apps and devices. They both recognized the importance of patience and sometimes required assistance from tech-savvy friends or family members.

Despite these challenges, the benefits outweighed the drawbacks. The technological aids provided a sense of independence and security. They could rely on reminders, stay engaged with brain training exercises, and even control their environment with smart home devices.

**Practical Advice**

Margaret, George, and Lisa's journey highlights several practical steps for those seeking to support their memory or mitigate dementia risk:

**1. Use a Dementia Risk Checklist:** Identify personal risk factors and take proactive steps to address them through lifestyle changes and regular health check-ups.

**2. Incorporate Memory Aids:** Utilize memory boards, memory books, and flashcards tailored to your specific needs and preferences.

**3. Embrace Technology:** Explore apps and devices that offer cognitive exercises and practical daily reminders. Seek help if needed to overcome initial learning curves.

By integrating these tools and techniques, individuals can take meaningful steps toward preserving their cognitive health and enhancing their quality of life. The journey of Margaret, George, and Lisa serves as a testament to the power of proactive measures and the support of both traditional and modern aids in navigating the complexities of memory and aging.

# CHAPTER 4

## EMERGENCY PREPAREDNESS: A COMPREHENSIVE GUIDE

Imagine you're a nurse, and the clock shows 2:00 AM in the emergency room. The doors swing open, and paramedics wheel in a patient. She's unconscious, and the only clue you have to her medical history is a crumpled piece of paper in her pocket. This scene underscores the importance of having a comprehensive and up-to-date medication list and medical history readily accessible.

**What to Include on a Medication List**

A good medication list is a lifeline. It should be clear, concise, and comprehensive. Here's what it should include:

- Prescription Medications: Name, dosage, frequency, and the prescribing doctor's name.
- Over-the-Counter Medications: Include everything from pain relievers to supplements.
- Allergies: List all known allergies, especially to medications.
- Adverse Reactions: Any past adverse reactions to medications should be noted.
- Immunizations: Dates and types of immunizations received.

Let's take an example: Jane, a 65-year-old with diabetes, hypertension, and a history of heart attacks. Her medication list might look like this:

- Metformin: 500 mg, twice daily, prescribed by Dr. Smith.

- Lisinopril: 20 mg, once daily, prescribed by Dr. Johnson.
- Aspirin: 81 mg, once daily, over-the-counter.
- Allergies: Penicillin (severe rash), Sulfa drugs (hives).

**Listing Physical Ailments and Medical History**

Equally important is a detailed record of physical ailments and medical history. This history provides context for the medication list and helps medical personnel make informed decisions. Key points to include:

- Chronic Conditions: Diabetes, hypertension, asthma, etc.
- Past Surgeries: Types of surgeries and dates.
- Hospitalizations: Reasons and dates.
- Family Medical History: Any hereditary conditions.
- Recent Tests: Results from blood tests, MRIs, etc.

Continuing with Jane's example, her medical history might include:

- Chronic Conditions: Type 2 diabetes (diagnosed 2005), hypertension (diagnosed 2010), history of myocardial infarction (2018).
- Surgeries: Appendectomy (1995), coronary artery bypass grafting (2018).
- Hospitalizations: Admitted for heart attack (2018).

**Creating an Emergency Plan**

Imagine you're in a crowded mall, and suddenly, you feel dizzy. Your vision blurs, and you know you're about to faint. In such moments, having a well-thought-out emergency plan can make all the difference.

**Steps to Prepare for Medical Emergencies**

**1. Assess Risks:** Identify potential health emergencies based on your medical history.

**2. Compile Essential Information:** Create a comprehensive medication list and medical history.

**3. Prepare an Emergency Kit:** Include medications, medical supplies (like a glucose meter for diabetics), a list of emergency contacts, and important documents.

**4. Educate Yourself:** Learn basic first aid and CPR.

**5. Inform Family and Friends:** Make sure they know about your medical conditions and how to respond in an emergency.

**Communication Strategies with Emergency Responders**

Clear communication can save lives. In an emergency, time is of the essence. Here's how to ensure effective communication:

- Wear a Medical ID: A bracelet or necklace that lists your key medical conditions and allergies.

- Use Technology: Apps like ICE (In Case of Emergency) can store medical information and can be accessed even if your phone is locked.
- Prepare a "Grab and Go" Bag: Keep a bag with essential items and documents ready at all times.

**Legal Documents**

In the midst of an emergency, legal documents can provide clarity and ensure your wishes are respected. Picture this: a patient is in critical condition, and the family is unsure about his wishes regarding life support. The presence of legal documents can guide the medical team and alleviate family stress.

**Importance of Having Legal Documents in Place**

Legal documents are the anchors in the tempest—power of attorney, advance directives, and healthcare proxies. They speak for us when words fail, ensuring wishes are honored and decisions aligned with our values. For Anna, whose father battled Parkinson's disease, these documents offered clarity amidst uncertainty, guiding medical decisions in line with his fervently expressed desires. Legal documents are crucial for several reasons:

- Ensuring Your Wishes Are Followed: They provide clear instructions for medical personnel and family members.
- Reducing Stress: They alleviate the burden on family members during critical moments.
- Preventing Disputes: Clear documentation can prevent potential conflicts among family members.

## How to Prepare and Store These Documents

Preparation begins with conversation—discussing wishes openly with loved ones and legal counsel. Documents should be clear, signed, and accessible: copies stored securely at home, with trusted family members, and in the care of legal advisors. In emergencies, their swift retrieval can turn chaos into coordinated care—a testament to foresight and preparation. Here's a practical guide to preparing and storing essential legal documents:

**1. Advance Directives:** Includes living wills and durable power of attorney for healthcare.

- Living Will: Specifies your wishes regarding medical treatments if you're unable to communicate.
- Durable Power of Attorney for Healthcare: Designates a person to make medical decisions on your behalf.

**2. Do Not Resuscitate (DNR) Orders:** Indicates your preference not to undergo CPR.

**3. Organ Donation Preferences:** Specifies whether you wish to donate your organs.

**Storage Tips:**

- Accessible Locations: Keep copies in a place that's easy to access, like a safe but reachable drawer.
- Digital Copies: Store digital versions on a secure cloud service.
- Inform Key People: Ensure family members and your designated healthcare proxy know where to find these documents.

In summary, emergency preparedness is not just about having a plan; it's about having the right information, communicating effectively, and ensuring your legal wishes are documented and accessible. By taking these steps, you can provide crucial guidance to medical personnel and peace of mind to yourself and your loved ones. So, take action today—prepare, communicate, and document to face emergencies with confidence and clarity.

# CHAPTER 5

## DISTRACTION TECHNIQUES FOR CAREGIVERS

Caring for someone with dementia or other cognitive impairments often involves navigating challenging behaviors and agitation. One effective approach to managing these moments is through distraction techniques that can soothe and engage the individual. Here, we explore several methods that caregivers can use, focusing on using nursery rhymes, the comfort of warm blankets, the role of food, and other sensory distractions.

**The Role of Music in Dementia Care**

Music has a profound impact on individuals with dementia. It can tap into deep-seated memories and emotions, often more effectively than words. Studies have shown that music can reduce agitation, improve mood, and even enhance cognitive function in dementia patients. The rhythmic and repetitive nature of nursery rhymes makes them particularly effective. Music is a timeless melody that transcends the barriers of memory and time. In the realm of dementia care, it becomes a lifeline—a bridge to moments of clarity and connection. Nursery rhymes, with their rhythmic cadence and familiar melodies, evoke echoes of childhood, stirring emotions that bypass the fog of forgetting. For Maria, whose mother found solace in "Twinkle, Twinkle, Little Star," these melodies became a beacon, guiding them through the maze of Alzheimer's.

**Examples of Effective Nursery Rhymes**

From "Row, Row, Row Your Boat" to "The Itsy Bitsy Spider," nursery rhymes offer simplicity wrapped in familiarity. Their repetitive nature and catchy tunes soothe restlessness, inviting participation and sparking memories thought lost. For caregivers, these rhymes become tools of engagement—opening doors to shared moments and smiles amid uncertainty.

1. **"Twinkle, Twinkle, Little Star"**- This timeless rhyme is soothing and familiar, often triggering positive memories from childhood.

2. **"You Are My Sunshine"**- A gentle, uplifting song that can brighten a patient's mood and provide a sense of comfort.

3. **"Baa Baa Black Sheep"**- The repetitive nature of this rhyme can be calming and reassuring.

4. **"Row, Row, Row Your Boat"**- The simple, repetitive lyrics can engage patients and encourage them to sing along.

**The Comfort of Warm Blankets**

**Sensory Techniques for Soothing Agitation**

Sensory stimulation is a powerful tool in dementia care. Warm blankets can provide physical comfort and a sense of security. The warmth can relax tense muscles and reduce anxiety, helping to calm agitated behaviors. This technique is particularly effective when combined with a gentle touch or a soothing voice. In the language of caregiving, warmth speaks volumes. Soft blankets, with their gentle embrace, offer more than physical comfort—they whisper reassurance, cocooning in safety and familiarity. For James, who faced moments of agitation with Alzheimer's, a cozy blanket became his sanctuary—a tangible reminder of care and security amidst the storm.

**Choosing the Right Materials**

Selecting blankets is an art of texture and touch. Opt for soft fabrics like fleece or cotton, soothing to sensitive skin. Consider weight too—a gentle pressure can provide a grounding effect, calming restlessness and easing anxiety. In the symphony of caregiving, these blankets compose notes of comfort, harmonizing with the rhythm of care.

When selecting blankets, consider the following:

- Softness: Choose blankets made from soft, non-irritating materials like fleece or cotton.
- Weight: Weighted blankets can provide additional sensory input and comfort.
- Temperature Regulation: Opt for materials that provide warmth without causing overheating.

**The Role of Food in Distraction and Comfort**

**Using Favorite Foods to Calm and Engage**

Food can be a powerful distraction and a source of comfort. The act of eating engages multiple senses, and favorite foods can evoke pleasant memories and feelings. Caregivers can use mealtimes as opportunities to distract and soothe their loved ones. Food is more than sustenance—it's a taste of memories, a journey through flavors that resonate deep within. In dementia care, favorite foods become portals to joy and engagement. From warm soups that stir the senses to familiar desserts that evoke smiles, these culinary comforts weave stories of connection. Recipes like chicken soup or apple pie evoke nostalgia, stirring reminiscences even when words falter.

**Recipes and Snack Ideas for Dementia Patients**

Consider crafting simple, nutritious meals tailored to personal tastes. A bowl of creamy oatmeal with berries for breakfast, or a plate of grilled cheese with tomato soup for lunch, can awaken appetites and foster moments of shared enjoyment. Snack ideas like sliced fruit or yogurt parfaits provide healthy indulgences, inviting participation in the pleasures of taste and texture.

**1. Smoothies:** Easy to consume and customizable, smoothies can be made with fruits, vegetables, and protein sources.

**2. Finger Foods:** Bite-sized snacks like cheese cubes, apple slices, or crackers are easy to handle and eat.

**3. Comfort Foods:** Familiar dishes like mashed potatoes, chicken soup, or oatmeal can be both nourishing and comforting.

**Other Distraction Techniques**

Beyond music and blankets lie a tapestry of sensory delights. Aromatherapy, with scents like lavender or peppermint, can calm and center. Tactile objects—smooth stones or textured fabrics—offer tangible connections, grounding in the present moment. Activities like simple puzzles or crafting projects engage hands and minds, nurturing creativity and focus amid the ebb and flow of caregiving.

**Aromatherapy, Tactile Objects, and More**

In addition to music, warm blankets, and food, there are numerous other distraction techniques that caregivers can employ:

- Aromatherapy: Scents like lavender, vanilla, and chamomile can have a calming effect. Essential oils or scented candles can be used to create a soothing environment.
- Tactile Objects: Items with interesting textures, such as soft toys, stress balls, or textured fabrics, can provide sensory stimulation and distraction.
- Storytelling: Sharing stories, whether from books or personal memories, can engage and comfort patients. Tailor the stories to their interests and past experiences.
- Visual Stimulation: Watching nature videos, looking at photo albums, or even observing fish in an aquarium can provide a calming distraction.

Practical Advice for Caregivers

**1. Be Patient and Observant:** Each individual is unique, so it's important to pay attention to what techniques are most effective for your loved one.

**2. Create a Routine:** Consistency can be comforting. Try to incorporate distraction techniques into a daily routine to provide structure.

**3. Involve the Individual:** Whenever possible, involve the person in the activity. Sing along to nursery rhymes together, or let them help with simple food preparation tasks.

**4. Use a Multisensory Approach:** Combining different types of sensory stimulation (e.g., music and aromatherapy) can enhance the calming effect.

Distraction techniques in caregiving are like gentle breezes in a turbulent sea—nurturing moments of calm amidst life's storms. From nursery rhymes that echo through generations to blankets that offer warmth and security, each technique tells a story—a story of care, compassion, and connection. As caregivers navigate the complexities of dementia, these tools—modern yet timeless—become beacons of comfort, illuminating paths of understanding and solace. In these moments of distraction, we find not just respite but also the enduring power of presence and love.

Incorporating these distraction techniques into daily care routines can significantly improve the quality of life for individuals with dementia and provide caregivers with effective tools to manage challenging behaviors.

# CHAPTER 6

## FOSTERING STRONG CONNECTIONS WITH DEMENTIA PATIENTS

Empathy is the cornerstone of caregiving for dementia patients. It goes beyond merely understanding the clinical aspects of the condition; it's about feeling the emotional weight carried by those affected and responding with compassion. Dementia can rob individuals of their memories, their sense of self, and their ability to communicate. As caregivers, our role is to bridge this gap with empathy, creating a safe and nurturing environment. Empathy is a language of understanding that transcends words. It's the ability to step into another's world, to feel their emotions as if they were your own. For Sarah, whose father navigated Alzheimer's, empathy meant listening with patience, embracing his reality with compassion. In these moments, she discovered that empathy isn't just a skill but a bridge—a lifeline connecting hearts in the face of uncertainty.

Imagine Sarah, a dedicated caregiver, who begins each day by immersing herself in the world of the residents she cares for. She doesn't just perform her tasks; she engages with them on a deeply personal level. When Mr. Thompson, a former jazz musician, becomes agitated, Sarah doesn't rush to calm him down with medication. Instead, she sits beside him, gently humming a familiar tune from his past. His eyes light up, and for a moment, he is transported back to the vibrant days of his youth. This is the power of empathy in action.

**Stories of Successful Empathetic Approaches**

Empathy can transform the caregiving experience. Take the story of Emma, a woman living with advanced dementia, and her daughter, Lisa. Lisa noticed that her mother, who once loved gardening, seemed particularly distressed during afternoons. Instead of focusing solely on managing the distress, Lisa began taking Emma to a nearby park every afternoon. They would walk slowly, smelling the flowers and feeling the sun on their faces. These moments brought peace to Emma and allowed Lisa to connect with her mother in a profound way.

Another example is Jack, a man with early-stage dementia, whose memories of fishing with his father were slipping away. His caregiver, Tom, arranged a small fishing trip. They didn't catch much, but the familiar activity brought a sense of normalcy and joy to Jack. This act of empathy not only alleviated Jack's anxiety but also fostered a strong bond between him and Tom.

**Supporting Family Members with Dementia**

Living with dementia is a journey of courage and adaptation—a path where roles shift and memories flicker. For families, it's a symphony of challenges and resilience, navigating each day with patience and love. Practical support—like establishing routines, ensuring safety, and seeking respite—becomes pillars of stability in the storm. Together, families learn to dance with dementia's rhythms, finding strength in unity and understanding.

Living with a family member who has dementia is both a challenge and a labor of love. It requires patience, resilience, and an abundance of support. Families often find themselves navigating uncharted waters, unsure of how to maintain their relationship with their loved one while managing the practical aspects of caregiving.

One crucial aspect is maintaining a routine. Routines provide a sense of stability and predictability, which can be incredibly comforting for someone with dementia. Simple activities like sharing meals, going for walks, or listening to music together can foster a sense of normalcy and connection.

### Navigating Family Dynamics and Roles

In the tapestry of family dynamics, roles evolve. Siblings become caregivers, children become advocates, and spouses become anchors in the storm. Communication—open, honest, and compassionate—guides these relationships, fostering unity amid uncertainty. For Anna's family, whose father faced dementia, shared responsibilities and mutual support became their compass, guiding them through uncharted waters with resilience and grace.

Dementia can strain family dynamics, as roles shift and responsibilities increase. Open communication is essential to ensure that everyone feels supported and heard. Families might consider regular meetings to discuss the caregiving process, share their feelings, and plan for the future.

Consider the story of the Martinez family. When their patriarch, Jorge, was diagnosed with dementia, his children initially struggled with the changes. They each had different ideas about his care. To navigate these dynamics, they began holding weekly family meetings, facilitated by a social worker. These sessions allowed them to express their concerns, delegate responsibilities, and support each other emotionally. Over time, they found a rhythm that worked for everyone, ensuring that Jorge received the best possible care while maintaining family harmony.

**Techniques to Foster Strong Connections**

Consider activities that stimulate the senses and ignite memories. Cooking together—a shared recipe passed down through generations—can evoke nostalgia and foster collaboration. Outdoor walks amidst nature's splendor offer moments of serenity and connection. Even simple games or puzzles can stimulate cognition and laughter, cultivating joy in shared experiences. Here are some techniques that have proven effective:

**1. Personalized Activities:** Tailor activities to the individual's interests and past experiences. Whether it's painting, baking, or listening to music, engaging in familiar activities can evoke positive emotions and memories.

**2. Memory Boxes:** Create a memory box filled with items that hold significance to the person. Photographs, trinkets, and letters can prompt conversations and trigger cherished memories.

**3. Sensory Stimulation:** Use sensory activities to engage different parts of the brain. Aromatherapy, tactile objects, and nature sounds can provide comfort and stimulate the senses.

**Activities That Promote Bonding**

Consider activities that stimulate the senses and ignite memories. Cooking together—a shared recipe passed down through generations—can evoke nostalgia and foster collaboration. Outdoor walks amidst nature's splendor offer moments of serenity and connection. Even simple games or puzzles can stimulate cognition and laughter, cultivating joy in shared experiences. Activities that promote bonding are invaluable in creating meaningful connections. Here are a few ideas:

**1. Storytelling:** Encourage storytelling sessions where the person can share their life experiences. Even if their memory is fragmented, the act of storytelling can be incredibly therapeutic.

**2. Art and Craft:** Engage in simple art and craft activities. Painting, knitting, or scrapbooking can be relaxing and provide a sense of accomplishment.

**3. Music Therapy:** Music has a profound impact on people with dementia. Playing their favorite songs or even having a little dance can uplift their spirits and create joyous moments.

**Communication Strategies**

Communication is a dance—a symphony of words and gestures that speak volumes. Speak slowly and clearly, using simple sentences and familiar words. Maintain eye contact and offer reassuring touches—a hand on the shoulder or a gentle squeeze—to convey warmth and understanding. Non-verbal cues—like smiles, nods, and facial expressions—bridge gaps in language, fostering connection beyond words. Effective communication with dementia patients requires sensitivity and adaptability. Here are some tips:

**1. Speak Clearly and Calmly:** Use simple, short sentences and speak slowly. Maintain eye contact and use a gentle tone.

**2. Non-Verbal Cues:** Pay attention to body language, facial expressions, and gestures. Sometimes, a smile or a reassuring touch can convey more than words.

**3. Active Listening:** Show that you are listening by nodding, maintaining eye contact, and responding appropriately. This encourages the person to express themselves.

**Encouraging Meaningful Conversation**

Encourage conversation that celebrates life's tapestry. Share stories of cherished memories, asking open-ended questions that invite reflection and storytelling. Validate emotions and listen actively, embracing their perspective with empathy and respect. In these moments, communication transcends dialogue—it becomes a testament to presence and love, weaving threads of connection that endure. Encouraging meaningful conversation can be challenging but is essential for maintaining a connection. Here are some strategies:

**1. Ask Open-Ended** Questions: Instead of yes/no questions, ask open-ended ones that encourage elaboration. For example, "Tell me about your favorite holiday."

**2. Validate Feelings:** Acknowledge their emotions, even if their words don't make complete sense. Saying, "I can see that you're upset. I'm here for you," can provide comfort.

**3. Use Reminiscence Therapy:** Engage in reminiscence therapy by discussing past events, looking at old photos, or listening to music from their youth. This can stimulate memories and facilitate meaningful conversation.

Fostering strong connections with dementia patients is a multifaceted and deeply rewarding endeavor. By understanding and empathizing, supporting family members, building connections, and employing effective communication strategies, caregivers can create an environment of love, respect, and dignity. It's about seeing beyond the condition and recognizing the person within, cherishing the moments of joy and connection that make the caregiving journey worthwhile. Fostering strong connections with dementia patients is a journey of empathy, understanding, and resilience. From empathetic caregiving that embraces their reality to supporting family dynamics with patience and love, each element enriches the tapestry of caregiving. Through activities that spark joy and communication that bridges worlds, we cultivate bonds that transcend memory—a testament to the enduring power of connection and compassion. In these moments, we find not just caregiving but also a profound exchange of love and humanity.

# CHAPTER 7

## CAREGIVER WELLNESS

Being a caregiver is one of the most selfless and challenging roles one can take on. It demands immense emotional, physical, and mental strength. In this journey, caregivers often prioritize the needs of others over their own, which can lead to burnout. To sustain this noble path, it's crucial for caregivers to focus on their own wellness. This guide delves into relaxation techniques, reflection practices, physical health, and mental health support tailored for caregivers, incorporating storytelling elements, modern language, and practical advice.

**Mindfulness Exercises for Caregivers**

Mindfulness is a sanctuary—a place of peace amidst the whirlwind of caregiving. It's the practice of being present, of embracing each moment with awareness and acceptance. For Emily, whose days were a blur of caregiving for her mother with dementia, mindfulness became a lifeline. Through simple practices—like focused breathing or body scan meditations—she found moments of calm, grounding herself in the present amid uncertainty.

Imagine Sarah, a full-time caregiver for her aging mother. Each day is a whirlwind of activities, leaving her little time for herself. Sarah discovers mindfulness, a technique that helps her stay present and grounded.

**Practice:** Every morning, Sarah sets aside ten minutes to sit quietly. She focuses on her breath, noticing the rise and fall of her chest. When her mind wanders to the day's tasks, she gently brings her attention back to her breathing. This simple act of mindfulness helps Sarah start her day with a sense of calm and clarity.

**Tip:** Use apps like Headspace or Calm, which offer guided mindfulness exercises specifically designed for busy individuals.

**Guided Relaxation Practices**

Imagine a tranquil shore—the ebb and flow of waves echoing the rhythm of relaxation. Guided imagery offers caregivers a voyage to serenity, painting mental landscapes of peace and tranquility. Visualize a favorite place—a sunlit meadow or a quiet beach—and immerse yourself in its sights, sounds, and sensations. Guided relaxation scripts, with soothing voices and gentle prompts, guide caregivers through waves of tension, leaving them refreshed and renewed.

John, another caregiver, struggles with unwinding after a long day of caring for his disabled brother. He turns to guided relaxation practices to help him decompress.

**Practice:** At night, John listens to guided relaxation tracks. A soothing voice takes him through a journey, imagining himself in a serene forest or on a tranquil beach. These guided practices not only relax his body but also transport his mind away from daily stresses.

**Tip:** Explore resources on YouTube or platforms like Insight Timer for a variety of guided relaxation sessions.

**The Importance of Self-Reflection**

Self-reflection is a mirror—a window into the soul of caregiving. It's the art of pausing, of turning inward to examine thoughts, emotions, and experiences. Journaling prompts caregivers to explore their journey—the highs and lows, the joys and challenges. For Michael, journaling became a companion in his caregiving for his father. Through reflective writing, he unearthed insights and found solace in sharing his journey on paper—a testament to the power of introspection.

Emily, caring for her autistic son, realizes that she often feels overwhelmed and disconnected from her own emotions. She learns the power of self-reflection to reconnect with herself.

Emily begins to set aside time each week to reflect on her experiences. She sits in a quiet space, thinking about the week's challenges and triumphs. This practice helps her gain insights into her emotions and behaviors, fostering a deeper understanding of herself.

**Tip:** Self-reflection can be as simple as asking yourself questions like, "What did I do well this week?" or "What could I have handled differently?"

**Journaling Prompts and Exercises**

Start with simple prompts: "Today, I felt most challenged when..." or "A moment of joy I experienced..." Explore emotions openly, without judgment, allowing thoughts to flow freely. Reflect on personal growth and accomplishments, celebrating small victories along the way.

Mark, balancing caregiving with a full-time job, finds solace in journaling. It becomes his outlet for expressing emotions he struggles to voice.

**Practice:** Each night, Mark writes in his journal. He starts with prompts like, "Today, I felt proud of myself because..." or "The most challenging part of my day was...". This routine helps him process his feelings and reduce stress.

**Tip:** Keep a journal by your bedside and dedicate just five minutes each day to jot down your thoughts. Over time, you'll notice patterns and gain valuable insights into your emotional well-being.

**Exercise Routines for Busy Caregivers**

Physical health is the anchor—a cornerstone of caregiver wellness. Incorporate simple exercises into daily routines: stretching upon waking, taking brisk walks during breaks, or practicing yoga for flexibility and relaxation. Short bursts of activity—like stair climbing or dancing to favorite tunes—revitalize both body and mind, boosting energy and reducing stress.

Linda, who cares for her elderly father, often skips exercise due to lack of time. She learns that short, efficient workouts can fit into her hectic schedule.

**Practice:** Linda discovers high-intensity interval training (HIIT), which requires just 20 minutes a day. She follows online videos that guide her through quick but effective routines, helping her stay fit without a significant time investment.

**Tip:** Look for workout apps or online videos that offer short, guided routines. Even a brisk 10-minute walk can make a significant difference in your physical health.

**Nutrition Tips to Maintain Energy Levels**

Nutrition fuels the journey—a compass guiding caregivers through long days and nights. Prioritize balanced meals rich in fruits, vegetables, lean proteins, and whole grains. Keep healthy snacks—like nuts, yogurt, or fresh fruit—readily available for quick refueling. Stay hydrated with water throughout the day, replenishing energy reserves and supporting overall well-being.

David, a caregiver for his spouse with chronic illness, often relies on fast food due to time constraints. He realizes that proper nutrition is essential for maintaining his energy levels.

**Practice:** David starts meal prepping on weekends. He prepares healthy, balanced meals that he can quickly reheat during the week. He focuses on incorporating lean proteins, whole grains, and plenty of fruits and vegetables into his diet.

**Tip:** Plan your meals ahead of time and keep healthy snacks like nuts, fruits, and yogurt readily available. Hydration is also key – aim to drink plenty of water throughout the day.

**Recognizing Signs of Stress and Anxiety**

Caregiving is a marathon, not a sprint—yet stress and anxiety can loom on the horizon. Recognize warning signs: fatigue, irritability, changes in sleep patterns. Listen to your body and mind, acknowledging emotions without judgment. Reach out to support networks—friends, family, or support groups—to share experiences and seek guidance. Remember, it's okay to ask for help.

Jessica, overwhelmed by her caregiving duties, begins to notice signs of chronic stress: irritability, trouble sleeping, and constant fatigue. She learns to recognize these signs as red flags. When Jessica starts feeling overly anxious, she acknowledges her stress rather than ignoring it. She practices deep breathing exercises and reaches out to a friend for support.

Tip: Be mindful of changes in your mood, energy levels, and sleep patterns. These can be indicators of stress or anxiety that need to be addressed.

**Resources for Professional Help**

Professional support is a beacon—a lifeline in times of uncertainty. Seek guidance from healthcare providers, counselors, or therapists specializing in caregiver support. Online resources, like caregiver forums or telehealth services, offer accessibility and convenience. Consider respite care options to recharge and rejuvenate, ensuring sustainable caregiving practices.

Alex, caring for his father with Alzheimer's, feels isolated and overwhelmed. He seeks professional help and joins a support group for caregivers.

**Practice:** Alex finds a therapist who specializes in caregiver stress. He also attends weekly support group meetings where he connects with others facing similar challenges. These resources provide him with emotional support and practical advice.

**Tip:** Don't hesitate to seek professional help if you're feeling overwhelmed. Look for local support groups, therapy services, or online forums for caregivers. Resources like the National Alliance for Caregiving and Caregiver Action Network offer valuable support and information.

Caregiving is a demanding and rewarding journey. By incorporating relaxation techniques, reflection practices, physical health routines, and mental health support, caregivers can maintain their well-being and continue to provide the best care possible. Remember, taking care of yourself is not a luxury but a necessity. Your wellness is the foundation that allows you to care for others effectively.

# CHAPTER 8

## AVOIDING CAREGIVER BURNOUT

Caring for a loved one can be incredibly rewarding, but it can also be a source of intense stress and exhaustion. Many caregivers give in to burnout because they are deeply committed to providing the best care possible, often neglecting their own needs in the process. Let's delve into why some caregivers succumb to burnout and the symptoms and warning signs to watch for.

**Why Some Caregivers Give in to Burnout**

Caregiving is a labor of love—a journey marked by dedication and compassion. Yet, amidst the noble calling, caregivers can find themselves at risk of burnout. The relentless demands of caregiving—emotional, physical, and logistical—can erode resilience over time. For Sarah, caring for her aging parents, burnout crept in slowly, disguised by her unwavering commitment. The weight of responsibility, coupled with the absence of self-care, cast shadows on her well-being, gradually dimming her light of resilience.

Imagine Sarah, a devoted daughter who took on the responsibility of caring for her elderly mother after a stroke. She juggles her job, household chores, and caregiving duties, convinced she can manage it all. Sarah is driven by love and a sense of duty, but she doesn't realize the toll it's taking on her health and well-being.

Caregivers like Sarah often give in to burnout because they underestimate the demands of caregiving and overestimate their capacity to handle everything alone. They might feel guilty about asking for help, believing they should be able to manage on their own. This self-imposed pressure, coupled with the emotional and physical demands of caregiving, can lead to burnout.

**Symptoms and Warning Signs**

Recognizing the symptoms of burnout is crucial for preventing it. Here are some common warning signs:

1. Physical Exhaustion: Constant fatigue that doesn't improve with rest.
2. Emotional Overwhelm: Feelings of helplessness, hopelessness, or being trapped.
3. Irritability and Anger: Becoming easily frustrated or angry over minor issues.
4. Withdrawal: Pulling away from social activities and isolating oneself.
5. Sleep Problems: Difficulty falling asleep or staying asleep, or sleeping too much.
6. Changes in Appetite: Eating too much or too little.
7. Health Issues: Frequent headaches, stomach problems, or other physical ailments.
8. Neglecting Personal Needs: Ignoring one's own health, hygiene, or well-being.

**Prevention Strategies**

Preventing burnout requires a mosaic of self-care practices woven into daily routines. Preventing caregiver burnout requires a proactive approach. Here are some tips and strategies to help you avoid burnout and maintain your well-being.

**Tips to Avoid Burnout**

1. Set Realistic Goals: Understand your limits and set achievable goals. Prioritize tasks and focus on what's most important.

2. Take Breaks: Schedule regular breaks throughout the day. Even a few minutes of downtime can make a big difference.

3. Practice Self-Care: Engage in activities that rejuvenate you, whether it's reading a book, going for a walk, or enjoying a hobby.

4. Stay Healthy: Maintain a balanced diet, exercise regularly, and get enough sleep. Your physical health is closely linked to your mental well-being.

5. Seek Professional Help: Don't hesitate to seek professional counseling or join a support group. Talking to others who understand your experience can be incredibly therapeutic.

6. Learn to Say No: It's okay to decline additional responsibilities or requests if you're already overwhelmed. Setting boundaries is essential.

**Building a Support Network**

A support network is a tapestry—a safety net of understanding and empathy. Cultivate connections with fellow caregivers, sharing experiences and insights through support groups or online forums. Seek guidance from healthcare professionals, counselors, or therapists specializing in caregiver support. Enlist family and friends in a shared caregiving journey, fostering collaboration and compassion. In unity, caregivers find strength—a collective shield against burnout's shadows. Building a support network is vital in preventing burnout. Here's how you can do it:

**1. Reach Out to Family and Friends:** Don't be afraid to ask for help from family members or friends. Even small tasks like running errands or preparing meals can lighten your load.

**2. Utilize Community Resources:** Look for local resources such as respite care services, adult day care centers, or volunteer organizations that offer assistance.

**3. Connect with Other Caregivers:** Join online forums or local support groups where you can share experiences and advice with other caregivers.

**4. Hire Professional Help:** If possible, consider hiring a professional caregiver to share the responsibilities. This can provide you with much-needed relief and peace of mind.

**Time Management**

Balancing caregiving with personal life can be challenging, but effective time management can help you achieve a healthier balance. Here are some strategies to manage your time efficiently.

**Balancing Caregiving with Personal Life**

Balancing caregiving with personal life is a tightrope walk—a delicate dance of priorities and boundaries. Start by setting realistic goals and establishing routines that accommodate both caregiving duties and personal needs. Break tasks into manageable steps, prioritizing essential responsibilities while delegating or postponing non-urgent tasks. Communicate openly with loved ones, setting clear expectations and seeking their support in navigating caregiving's ebbs and flows.

Imagine Mark, a father of two who also cares for his elderly father with dementia. He felt overwhelmed until he learned to balance his caregiving duties with his personal life. Here's how Mark manages it:

**1. Create a Schedule:** Mark creates a daily schedule that includes time for caregiving, work, family, and personal activities. This helps him stay organized and ensures he doesn't neglect any aspect of his life.

**2. Prioritize Tasks:** He identifies the most critical tasks each day and focuses on completing those first. This reduces the stress of feeling like everything needs to be done at once.

**3. Delegate Responsibilities:** Mark involves his family in caregiving tasks. His children help with household chores, and he enlists the help of a part-time caregiver for his father.

**Efficient Scheduling Techniques**

Efficient scheduling is a compass—a guide through the labyrinth of caregiving demands. Use calendars or apps to organize appointments, medications, and daily routines. Allocate time for self-care—whether it's exercise, relaxation, or social activities—to replenish energy reserves. Consider respite care options to recharge periodically, ensuring sustained resilience in caregiving. Flexibility is key—adjust schedules as needed to accommodate unforeseen challenges, embracing adaptability in the journey. To manage your time effectively, consider these scheduling techniques:

**1. Use a Planner:** Whether it's a physical planner or a digital app, keeping track of appointments, tasks, and reminders can help you stay organized.

**2. Set Alarms and Reminders:** Use alarms or notifications to remind you of important tasks and appointments.

**3. Time Blocking:** Allocate specific blocks of time for different activities. For example, dedicate mornings to caregiving tasks and afternoons to personal activities.

**4. Batch Tasks:** Group similar tasks together to save time and reduce the mental load of switching between activities.

**5. Review and Adjust:** Regularly review your schedule and make adjustments as needed. Flexibility is key to managing unexpected challenges.

Avoiding caregiver burnout is essential for maintaining your well-being and providing the best care possible for your loved one. By recognizing the symptoms of burnout, implementing prevention strategies, building a support network, and managing your time effectively, you can navigate the challenges of caregiving with resilience and grace. Remember, taking care of yourself is not a luxury—it's a necessity.

# CHAPTER 9

## FINANCIAL SAFEGUARDING

Financial safeguarding is a critical aspect of protecting and managing assets, especially for individuals diagnosed with dementia. This comprehensive guide will cover protecting finances, recognizing financial abuse and fraud, long-term financial planning, working with financial advisors, understanding insurance options, and navigating government benefits and programs.

**Tips to Safeguard the Finances of People Diagnosed with Dementia**

Emily had always been close to her father, John. When he was diagnosed with dementia, she knew she needed to take steps to protect his finances. Here's what she learned:

**1. Early Legal Arrangements:** Emily first arranged for a durable power of attorney (POA). This legal document allowed her to make financial decisions on John's behalf once he could no longer manage his affairs.

**Tip:** Establish a durable POA early, while the person with dementia can still make legal decisions.

**2. Simplify Finances:** Emily consolidated John's multiple bank accounts and investments into fewer, more manageable accounts.

**Tip:** Streamline finances to reduce complexity and ease management.

**3. Automatic Bill Payments:** To ensure that John's bills were paid on time, Emily set up automatic bill payments.

   **Tip:** Automate recurring payments to avoid missed deadlines and late fees.

**4. Monitor Accounts:** Emily regularly checked John's bank statements and credit reports for unusual activity.

   **Tip:** Frequently review financial statements to catch any irregularities early.

**5. Limit Cash Access:** Emily reduced the amount of cash John carried and limited his access to credit cards.

   **Tip:** Control cash flow and limit access to credit to prevent overspending or financial exploitation.

**Recognizing Financial Abuse and Fraud**

Mrs. Smith, an elderly woman with early-stage dementia, was almost tricked into giving her bank details to a scammer posing as a bank representative. Fortunately, her vigilant neighbor, Mr. Harris, intervened.

**1. Unusual Withdrawals:** Be alert to large or frequent withdrawals that are out of character.

   Warning Sign: Sudden, large sums of money being withdrawn or transferred.

**2. Strange Purchases:** Monitor for purchases that seem unusual for the individual's lifestyle.

   Warning Sign: Buying high-value items or services they wouldn't normally use.

**3. New Friends or Caregivers:** Be cautious of new acquaintances who quickly become overly involved in financial matters.

Warning Sign: New "friends" or caregivers who take a keen interest in the person's finances.

**4. Pressure to Change Legal Documents:** Be wary of anyone pushing the person to alter their will or other legal documents.

Warning Sign: Coercion to modify wills, powers of attorney, or beneficiary designations.

**Financial Planning**

**Long-term Financial Planning for Dementia Care**

The Thompsons faced a challenging journey when the family patriarch, Mr. Thompson, was diagnosed with dementia. They sought advice on how to plan for the long-term financial implications.

**1. Estimate Costs:** Understand the potential costs of dementia care, including in-home care, assisted living, and nursing home facilities.

Advice: Research the average costs of various care options in your area and plan accordingly.

**2. Budgeting:** Develop a comprehensive budget that accounts for current and future expenses.

Advice: Include medical expenses, caregiving costs, and everyday living expenses in your budget.

**3. Savings and Investments:** Evaluate savings and investment accounts to ensure they align with future care needs.

Advice: Consider shifting investments to more conservative options to preserve capital.

**4. Legal and Financial Documents:** Ensure all important documents, such as wills, trusts, and POAs, are up-to-date.

Advice: Regularly review and update legal documents to reflect current wishes and circumstances.

### Working with Financial Advisors

The Johnson family decided to seek professional help to navigate the complexities of dementia care finances.

**1. Find a Specialist:** Look for a financial advisor with experience in elder care and dementia planning.

Advice: Choose an advisor who understands the specific financial challenges associated with dementia.

**2. Regular Meetings:** Schedule regular check-ins with the financial advisor to adjust plans as needed.

Advice: Stay proactive and flexible, adapting the financial plan as circumstances change.

**3. Transparency:** Ensure clear communication between the advisor, the person with dementia, and their caregivers.

Advice: Maintain open and honest dialogue to make informed decisions.

## Understanding Insurance Options

Mary had always managed the household finances, but when her husband Alan was diagnosed with dementia, she realized they needed a solid understanding of their insurance options.

**1. Health Insurance:** Review health insurance policies to understand coverage for dementia care.

Advice: Know what your health insurance covers, including doctor visits, medications, and specialized treatments.

**2. Long-term Care Insurance:** Consider purchasing long-term care insurance to cover future care needs.

Advice: Investigate long-term care policies early, as premiums increase with age and health conditions.

**3. Disability Insurance:** Check if disability insurance policies can provide income if the person with dementia can no longer work.

Advice: Understand the terms and benefits of any disability insurance policies you hold.

**Navigating Government Benefits and Programs**

When the Lewises needed additional support for their mother's dementia care, they explored various government benefits and programs.

**1. Medicare:** Utilize Medicare benefits for medical care and prescription drugs.

  Advice: Ensure you understand Medicare's coverage limits and out-of-pocket costs.

**2. Medicaid:** Apply for Medicaid if eligible, to help cover long-term care costs.

  Advice: Medicaid can be a crucial resource for covering extensive care expenses, but eligibility requirements must be met.

**3. Social Security Disability Insurance (SSDI):** Explore SSDI if the person with dementia was employed and paid into Social Security.

Advice: SSDI can provide financial assistance to those who are no longer able to work due to disability.

**4. Veterans Benefits:** If the person with dementia is a veteran, investigate benefits through the Department of Veterans Affairs.

Advice: Veterans may be eligible for additional support and resources tailored to their needs.

By incorporating practical advice with relatable stories, this guide aims to provide a comprehensive understanding of financial safeguarding for individuals with dementia and their families. Taking these steps can help ensure that financial resources are protected and managed effectively, providing peace of mind during a challenging time.

# CHAPTER 10

## ENGAGING ACTIVITIES FOR DEMENTIA PATIENTS

Dementia can present challenges, but engaging activities can significantly enhance the quality of life for both patients and caregivers. Simple and fun activities tailored to their cognitive abilities are key. Here's a look at various activities and how to adapt them:

**Creative Activities to Do with Your Loved One:**

**1. Art Therapy:** Engage in painting, drawing, or crafting. Use simple supplies like watercolors or clay, focusing on the process rather than the outcome. Encourage creativity without pressure.

**2. Music Therapy:** Music can evoke memories and emotions. Listen to familiar songs, sing together, or play instruments like tambourines or simple percussion. Create playlists of favorite tunes from their youth.

**3. Storytelling and Reminiscing:** Encourage storytelling by discussing old photos, asking open-ended questions about their past, or creating a story together. Use prompts to guide conversations and keep them engaged.

**4. Gardening:** Tending to plants or a small garden can provide sensory stimulation and a sense of accomplishment. Choose easy-to-care-for plants and involve them in watering, planting seeds, or arranging flowers.

**Adapting Activities to Different Stages of Dementia:**

**Early Stage:** Focus on activities that stimulate memory and cognition, such as puzzles, word games, or baking simple recipes together. Maintain routines and encourage independence.

**Middle Stage:** Simplify tasks and activities, using visual cues and step-by-step instructions. Engage in activities that involve sensory stimulation, like aromatherapy, textured objects, or music.

**Late Stage:** Opt for activities that provide comfort and sensory experiences, such as gentle massage, listening to soothing music, or looking at photo albums. Focus on creating a calm and familiar environment.

**Physical Activities**

Physical activities are crucial for maintaining mobility, coordination, and overall well-being. Here are safe exercises suitable for dementia patients:

**1. Chair Exercises:** Seated exercises can include gentle stretches, leg lifts, and arm movements. Use music or storytelling elements to make it more engaging.

**2. Walking and Movement:** Take short walks in safe environments like gardens or quiet streets. Use verbal cues and simple instructions to guide them during walks.

**3. Dance Therapy:** Dancing to familiar tunes can improve mood and physical coordination. Choose slow-paced music and guide them through simple dance movements.

**4. Yoga and Tai Chi:** These gentle exercises promote relaxation and improve balance. Use clear demonstrations and verbal cues, incorporating storytelling elements to guide movements.

**Practical Advice**

- Patience and Flexibility: Understand that abilities may fluctuate daily. Be patient and adapt activities based on their current mood and cognitive state.
- Create a Calm Environment: Minimize distractions and noise to help them focus better on activities. Use soft lighting and comfortable seating arrangements.
- Encourage Social Interaction: Participate in activities together or involve other family members and friends. Social engagement can enhance their mood and provide a sense of belonging.

Engaging activities for dementia patients should be approached with sensitivity and tailored to their individual needs. By focusing on simple, enjoyable activities and adapting them as dementia progresses, caregivers can foster meaningful connections and improve the overall quality of life for their loved ones.

.

# CONCLUSION

## EMBRACING WISDOM AND HOPE

In concluding our journey through "Dementia Reflections," we reflect on the profound lessons learned and the enduring spirit that illuminates every page. This book has been more than a guide—it has been a companion, walking alongside caregivers, families, and individuals navigating the complexities of dementia care.

Throughout these pages, we have explored the depths of empathy and understanding, witnessing the transformative power of compassion in caregiving. We have delved into practical strategies for supporting loved ones, from memory aids and engaging activities to safeguarding finances and nurturing caregiver wellness. Each chapter has woven together stories of resilience, moments of connection, and the unwavering dedication that defines the journey of dementia care.

As we look back, we celebrate the courage of caregivers who face each day with grace and determination. We honor the strength of individuals living with dementia, whose spirits shine brightly even amidst the challenges. We acknowledge the importance of community and support networks, which provide solace and guidance in times of uncertainty.

"Dementia Reflections" is not just a book—it is a testament to the human spirit's capacity for growth, understanding, and hope. It reminds us that within every challenge lies an opportunity for compassion and learning, and that through empathy, we can create meaningful connections that transcend words.

As we close this chapter, may the reflections shared here continue to inspire and guide. May they serve as a beacon of wisdom and comfort for those embarking on their own journey with dementia. And may they reinforce our collective commitment to nurturing dignity, love, and resilience in every step of the way.

In embracing these reflections, we embrace the essence of caregiving—the profound journey of heart and soul that binds us all in a tapestry of compassion and understanding.

www.ingramcontent.com/pod-product-compliance
Lightning Source LLC
Chambersburg PA
CBHW062121220526
45471CB00010B/3823